Critical Praise for Felicia Luna Lemus

for *Like Son*

"Felicia Luna Lemus is a literary alchemist: she combines words that you never before thought could exist in the same sentence. She breaks all the rules and makes you wonder why you thought there were any. But enough about her style . . . The characters in *Like Son* are truly original creations—it would take a heart of stone not to love them."   —Vendela Vida, author of *The Diver's Clothes Lie Empty*

"*Like Son* is a love story that, like a psychic's trick, leaves nothing unbent: not gender, not culture north and south of the border, not time, or friendship, not even love itself. Don't try to understand how it happens; just watch, and be amazed."
                                        —Paul La Farge, author of *The Night Ocean*

"*Like Son* moves on the wings of a soulful, visceral kind of androgyny. Old men, young men, hot girls—all step forward and sing from their stuttering hearts. *Like Son* is one terrific read."
                                        —Eileen Myles, author of *Cool for You*

"Felicia Luna Lemus's fresh yet plain-spoken prose roots us in today's sad and sweeping chaos, as hope, love, and wild myth propel her unique characters into an unknown future. *Like Son* is a sweet song of a story."   —Michelle Tea, author of *Against Memoir*

"Chaos and fate are hopelessly intertwined in this exuberant second novel . . . Lemus doesn't waste a word in this smart, never sentimental novel."   —*Publishers Weekly*

"With prose that nearly sings off the page, Lemus [tells] an ancient story about love that's worth waiting for."   —*Out*

"[A] powerfully written chronicle of love." —*Booklist*

"Felicia Luna Lemus is a writer with a serious voice."
—*Time Out New York*

"The lyricism of [*Like Son*] swelled up and down my spine and gave me goose bumps . . . Lemus, I think, may be knocking on the door of greatness . . . I'll be waiting breathlessly to see what she does next." —*Lambda Book Report*

"A writer with an unparalleled literary style and attitude, Felicia Luna Lemus comes charging full force . . . *Like Son*, with its fluid prose and a narrative voice that always strikes the perfect pitch, demonstrates her fully realized skills as a novelist."
—*El Paso Times*

for *Trace Elements of Random Tea Parties*

"Outrageous and glorious . . . a wild ride worth every damn cent you spent for the ticket!"
—Helena María Viramontes, author of *Their Dogs Came with Them*

"A welcome contribution to Chicana letters from the new generation."
—Ana Castillo, author of *The Mixquiahuala Letters*

"Her sentences at their best are so condensed, so packed and hot, they're on the verge of exploding . . . Bursting at the seams with pizzazz and invention." —*San Francisco Chronicle*

"Edgy, exuberant . . . fun, rollicking and a little bit dangerous . . ."
—*Publishers Weekly*

"Lemus's dynamic language and pacing . . . offer deep insights into familia and cultura without an ounce of heavy-handedness."—*Latina*

PARTICULATE MATTER

FELICIA LUNA LEMUS

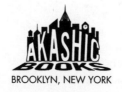

AKASHIC
BOOKS
BROOKLYN, NEW YORK

Published by Akashic Books
©2020 Felicia Luna Lemus

Author photo: Nina Revoyr
Cover art: "What Matters," Sonya Cheuse
Cover design: Sohrab Habibion

Hardcover ISBN: 978-1-61775-841-6
Library of Congress Control Number: 2020935821
First printing

Akashic Books
Brooklyn, New York
Twitter: @AkashicBooks
Facebook: AkashicBooks
E-mail: info@akashicbooks.com
Website: www.akashicbooks.com

Nina

Today is the longest day. Sun blazing, heavy thick solid air—purple mountains disappeared, downtown skyscrapers muted twinkle, observatory a dull smudge out west.

"It feels like my lungs are sunburned," you say.

We speed toward fluorescent lights and bleached floors and automatic sliding glass doors that open too goddamned slow.

Again.

My father's first wife died in a car accident, at his side, pregnant with the child I once, when I was a child myself, thought was the first me. When my father died, twenty-three years later, he left me his first wife's wedding rings.

You are the age he was when he died.

I push this thought from my mind.

The rings are jade and gold. They fit me perfectly.

A lightning bolt killed my great-grandfather. We are far from those rural fields now, one country north and in a city bigger than he ever saw. Doesn't matter. It was naive of me to think the skies could be neutral.

Hummingbird nest at our front gate. Hair of the dog. A few of mine, too: silver. Delicate twigs, tiny crawling rose leaves, and a bit of white thread. Tangled into the most beautiful little nest.

I put the nest in a ziplock, to freeze it (to sterilize it; quoth my mother, "All things die in the freezer," her collection of exquisite oddities stored beside ice cube trays), to keep it on my desk. Then the whole thing makes me sad, that empty fallen nest. I should put it back where I found it. But it's mine now.

Car full of things you need, I drive the long drive to the shore—to the little house, home-not-home, your new (temporary, I pray) residence, the place where you can breathe. Literally. I fold the hanging towels, mop the bathroom floor, rinse the tub, square the corners of every bottle and tube on the counters, gather empty dry-cleaner wire hangers and throw them in the blue bin. I don't even know if this town recycles like at home, our real home, home-home. Everything in its place [you are not].

The digital *Prepare to Stop* sign at the ramp from the 105 East to the 110 North homeward is malfunctioning, flashing wild rave style, no pattern discernable. The yellow *Slow* lights, too. Whoever hacked them gets bonus points for style. Slow, slow, slow . . .

[full stop]

Red-tailed hawks screech in the canyon all night.

I learn:

> They defend their nests something fierce.
>
> When mating, the female displays her talons in mock battle.
>
> They pair until death do them part.

I toss and turn, but I do not take your side of the bed.

Our anniversary, I unearth the embroidered wedding gift I made for you, packed away these seven years. I hang it in the little house kitchen.

Ruth 1:16–17.

And Ruth said, *Whither thou goest, I will go; and where thou lodgest, I will lodge.* [I cannot.]

El ala: wing, as in that which my ancients said propels the flight of a hummingbird from this world to the other.

La ola: wave, as in the ones we watch on our daily walk at the shore—searching for a sign, advice, assurance that this will get better, for a reminder of something larger than ourselves.

Ojalá: hopefully.

O Allah. From your lips to God's ears.

O$_3$. Nomenclature: from the Greek verb ὄζειν (*ozein* in Latin), "to smell."

Late night on the 110 North is chockablock full of straight-up psychos.

And the honking. Why the honking in tunnels? 110 to the 5 (or off at Fig). Three tunnels in a row. And the hairpin turn onto the 5—dear lord, people, slow the fuck down.

One car space for every 10 mph . . . my father taught me that.

I turn off the radio. Focus. Stretch my hands one at a time, cramped from my grip.

Cars cut me off, close the gap between home and me.

The dog's Frisbee flew into the living room floor lamp—the leaning, wobbly lamp closest the bedroom door. Ripped a hole straight through the lampshade and stayed there, neon orange and blue jutting out from beige. The impact turned the light on and knocked the three-level-brightness wiring back into working order. But the lampshade is torn beyond repair.

I never liked that lamp very much. Did you?

Fireworks, late at night and a week too soon. Doesn't anyone else think this sounds like war?

Wednesdays are senior discount day at the car wash.
Waiting room for heaven, hell of a wait.

Over at the bumper-sticker-car hippie house, a woman I've never seen before got out of a blue car holding a triangle American flag. I want to know where she put it.

When I was a kid, the folded flag was on the piano bench. I undid the first (last) origami tuck once. I wanted to unfurl the entire thing, shake it out and wrap myself in it, hide, disappear. Because that's what happens. People disappear in those dense triangles, their weight the totality of a human life.

It's cooled down at night for the first time in weeks. The moon is waxing. I almost believe this summer will end someday.

Explosions, machine-gun rounds, fires.

Something in the little house is no good, makes your lungs burn. New cabinets? Paint? The laminate floors? Coastal air, that remains good. And so you set up a tent in the backyard every night to sleep. You don't tell me about the rat that falls out of the tree and onto the tent. I only know about the squirrels eating peaches in sunlight.

The tiny ants in the backyard there are mean, aggressive, biting little fucks. I've never hated ants before. I do now.

The flying beetle with the luminescent-green body buzzed and chased us indoors.

Amelia Earhart's plane was an Electra.

Woke coughing. The sky heavy with ash and smoke. No mandatory evacuations for our area, but that air is here now.

City crews showed up this morning, a massive truck right outside the gate when I took the dog out. Other trucks clog the road, block my car in. Drills and bulldozers rip up asphalt. Everything loud, hectic, a total mess.

Bomb scare at your office. Downtown tower on lockdown.

Shooting death at the freeway exit I'll take tonight to see you.

Inhale, exhale, I focus on my breath.

The time that one guru snapped at her assistants when her flesh-tone headset microphone kept malfunctioning. Sitting lotus on the yoga studio platform, white dress billowing out around her, blond hair flowing hot-iron curls, eyes on fire.

That was awesome.

Murder of crows. Hawks screeching. Night-blooming cactus.

My One.

I love your sincerity.

I *miss* you.

"We're becoming beach people."

[Neither of us really believes this.]

Optics.

Tattoos and orthotics.

The woman at the register in the fancy house stuff store in the new (temporary) neighborhood makes me open the trashcan I buy for home-not-home, to prove I haven't tried to steal anything. She does this with a pleased smile. "Now there's nothing inside that, right?" she says. I smile my best deadeye kill-you-with-kindness smile, likely the second smile I ever learned, right after genuine joy. "Of course not, see?" I say.

The young woman at Starbucks in the new (temporary) neighborhood asks for my name and then says, "Oh, you're going to have to spell that one for me." Her smile coded like I'm beginning to realize might be standard issue here. Her marker and dirty cash register fingers touch the lip of my cup. "Sure, no problem," I say, my best second smile . . .

"F," as in . . . *do not try me,*
"E," as in *Eugene, my father, great-grandson of the ambassador of exports to the king of Sweden, Flemish on his other side and in the surname that once was my hyphenate,*
"L," as in *Luna, family name of my native blood, name of the moon in the sky,*
"I," as in *indigenous, Chichimeca, nomadic, here now and always, you will not lord over me, this land is not yours, you cannot steal what cannot be owned,*
"C," as in . . . *I will not say it,*
"I," *I will not repeat myself,*
"A," as in

My God, just give me the cup of tea already.

Chicanery.

Indian giver.

Going Dutch.

Gypped.

(For one stupid moment in time, long ago, I thought we'd gotten post-all-of-this, all of us.)

Don't they have an app for that?

It has been two months, my love. Two months of not once sleeping in the same bed, you sleeping in no bed at all, this I drive back home every night to take care of home, our dog, this I wake with you not, this you can't come home, this "home" that was once our forever home and will never be our home again.

Midday, a coyote runs past the house. Not the handsome pup I saw last night when I drove up the hill, as I closed the daily loop from the shore. Not the one with caution in his step. This one older, railish, rough patches of fur. No fear in his stride.

Mourning dove on the wire. Hummer at the cactus. Mockingbirds in the canyon. Squirrel in the walnut tree. Hens in the neighbor's coop. The dog across the canyon. Something rustling through the fallen rubber tree leaves in the extra lot.

Tender buttons.

Give me winter under cultivation.

Helicopter overhead. Jackhammer out front. Deep rumble city trucks stalled. In my chest. My bones. Every nerve and breath.

The firefighter's children across the canyon only need spears and to chant, "Kill the pig."

Goddamned jackhammers.

I should probably stop scowling at people so often.

For years I've thought my sunglasses were opaque. They are not.

"You are the most beautiful sight I've ever seen," I say,
the daughter of the blind man.

Home is where the heart is. A family meal feeds the soul. Home Sweet Home. Apple crisp.

I loved Home Ec. That was seventh grade.

This bean and cheese burrito is, as always, too much for me to eat. Your half is waiting for you.

Pan dulce. Elotes. Yolk-yellow sugared dough tucked inside. I know which market has the best ones. One either knows already or doesn't.

The hearing in my right ear keeps going out, quiet whispers. I stand at the mirror and hold a flashlight to my ear. The whispers stop.

Flashlight to my ear, a tiny spider crawled out toward the light. The loud scratching only I could hear stopped. (I was sixteen that time.)

I wake with a brown widow bite on the back of my leg. One red dot and two red branches of venom coursing through my veins. This is how I get superpowers, right? Either this or I fall into a vat of something toxic.

I keep walking into spiderwebs face-first.

Another web.

A neighbor keeps finding scorpions in her house. Maybe from the trees in the canyon the other neighbor cut down, she says. I tell her about my brown widow bite. She is unimpressed.

"A *scorpion* stung me as I slept," she says.

"I'm a Scorpio," she says.

Oh.

(I am not.)

The doorbell rings, late at night. Nobody is there. It rings again. And again. Nobody. I check for spider-webs. (The electrician showed me that the time the smoke detector wouldn't stop.)

Nothing.

Seriously, what the fuck?

I am beyond exhausted and numb.

I don't want to get used to this.

Note to crossword: contractions and word clusters are cheating.

It's been a day and still I'm bothered.

Late-night QVC is pure opium. The "Christmas in July" flameless candles and the jewelry are my favorites. Okay, and the mineral makeup close-ups and the shower gel demonstrations with the shower puffs in the clear glass kitchen bowls, too. But not the housewares or garden supplies or celebrity lines. Honestly, the call-in testimonials alone are plenty. I've never actually bought anything. I just watch. How do the hosts get their nails like that, like mannequin hands?

Tradecraft.

We settle in on the front porch, camping chairs our theater seats, my iPad our screen. The movie you've been telling me about, the one with the actor from the other movie you love so much, the one I've never been able to totally understand, all baseball glory and boy nostalgia, the movie I know I would weep to watch if ever you were gone. The actor is young in this movie. He is dashing in his Navy officer uniform. He is a spy, it turns out. That would be good enough. But there's also: the femme fatale from the other movie, the one I love with the dystopic metropolitan future and origami silver unicorn, the movie you've never understood the appeal of but that I like to think would make you weep to watch if ever I was gone.

That was the most delicious spy movie date.

My sweet Spy Baby.

Down the rabbit hole we go.

Metiche.

Chismosa.

Escandalosa.

Greñuda.

Ni modo.

That ten-minute nap with you on the new bed. Heaven.

[I hope we can keep it.]

That cup of peppermint tea you made for me with a spoonful of wildflower honey. Heaven.

You. Heaven.

The clouds there almost look like something tonight.

It drizzled here. Faker thunderstorm. Never came.

Godfingers: those rays of light reaching out from behind the clouds.

"I only love simplicity. I have a horror of pretense."
—Saint Thérèse, "The Little Flower" of Lisieux,
age twenty-four, on her deathbed

[I smelled roses. There were no roses.]

Jolie laide.

Wabi-sabi.

And now home-not-home has a couch. Used and ugly as hell, a soft place to land.

The millennial neighbor at Coyote Canyon spent thousands on landscaping, but still has flattened cardboard boxes for window dressing.

Why are people who canvas with petitions to save the canyon always Charles Mansons in crimson-red waxed sedans?

I've become the person who gives stink-eye while walking the dog when drivers don't come to a full stop at the corner.

I smell fire. There is no fire. I read somewhere once that this can be a sign of a brain tumor. I don't have a brain tumor. I call the dog in, shut all the windows.

I'm good at mirrors. Smoke, not at all.

It's impossible to photograph the moon with my phone.
I respect her for that.

European paper wasps. At least fifty of them. High in the sky like a pizza pie. Under the awning where the small triangle panel flew off years ago. They swoop as I water plants in the side yard.

Praying mantis at the pink room door. Sat with me all afternoon as I worked. And was on the screen door this morning, too. He's gone now.

I am the champion of the crossword today. Where is my trophy?

The dog ate black walnuts from under the rubber tree in the side yard. Rotted and poison and how did we not know this? She's sicker than I told you. I don't want you to worry. I'll take her to the vet if she needs to go. This knowing when to go to the doctor, how to take care like a doctor until that point, this is my second nature, my first books Harvard medical textbooks, highlighted and illustrated with my Crayons. Our girl, she's sick. But she will be okay.

I chop down the walnut tree.

[Someone else does it, but it is done.]

The neighbor tells me about the raccoon that chased him in their yard. As he talks—hand to mouth, hand to mouth several times—he eats. "Do you have a walnut tree?" he asks. "We did." He eats more. Maybe nothing bad will happen to him. He didn't have the walnuts when the raccoon chased him. That was a week ago.

If we can't stay (you already can't), I'll miss the lemon tree.

Hold a flashlight up to this and you'll see my secret message written just for you.*

*Lemon juice from our tree was my ink.

I was always the kid who had my page all strange diagonal on the desk in front of me, hunched over it super intense, obsessed with getting cursive just right, pressing down on the pencil so hard the point broke nearly every word, callus on the inside of my middle finger and under my thumb from steady pressure.

I learned then to take the page I've written on and the page underneath it, too.

I don't want anyone to rub a pencil across traces of etched imprint and see what isn't for them.

In eighth grade I learned how to read palms. It was equal parts lines and lines—on the palm and spoken. I memorized a generic script in one of those Time-Life *Mysteries of the Unknown* books and faked my way through the rest. Reading people, micro-gestures and all, came easy to me. Same for figuring out what people want to hear. It leaves me empty and anxious and unmoored, but I'm damn good at fortune-telling.

Macabre.

Macramé.

The nursery sells decorative nets for hanging plants. Thick twine, rough to the touch, braided from another era. I carry one around the store while we shop, its wooden beads ground me as a rosary might some. I put it back before we buy the plants you read can clean inside air.

Chlorophytum comosum. Commonly known as "spider plant."

The evening air is witchy cool. I sweep the patio and then wash my broom.

Record-breaking heat wave.

The grass is going to die. All the jade, too. The lemon tree, avocado tree, and night-blooming cacti will live. They've survived world wars.

Breathtaking Technicolor sunset. (Smog.)

Indian summer.

Dog days.

The Great Horned Owls have returned, flirting at each other come dusk. Not their usual spot on the telephone poles out front. Coyote Canyon.

I smell fire again.

Half past midnight, I see the flames. I gather what matters. Dog crate in car, leash, wallet, keys at the door. Our computers. The photo my dad took of little kid me standing on the roof, his hat shading my eyes, smart little smile, swag to my stance, that easy joy and confidence I'm always trying to find again. Three wooden urns in a duffle (the irony of packing ashes not lost on me). Your little kid album, red. My baby album, floral blue. Our courting correspondences you printed out and gave me on our first, paper, anniversary. Our wedding album.

One in the morning, I text you, hose down the yard and the fence.

Five thousand acres and growing.

Ash falls like light snow, caught in my lashes, in my breath, the sun gray.

Ten percent contained. A shift in the winds, it could ignite all over again.

Three months.

Four.

"I'm writing a book," I say.
"Is it fiction or nonfiction?" you ask.
"Yes."

Five.

And six.

"It needs an ending," you say.
"Yes."

[There is no end in sight.]

Acknowledgments

Thank you Johnny Temple, Johanna Ingalls, Aaron Petrovich, Ibrahim Ahmad, and the entire Akashic team. You're amazing, and I'm honored to work with you again.

Ariat Luna, sweet wild one, thank you for your love, for all that you teach me and for the laughter and comfort you bring. Meditation breaks, cookies and cuddles forever and ever.

Nina Revoyr. Thank you for your love, for the inspiration of your brilliance, for your profound kindness, beauty and strength. It will take an eternity to express how much I love you. In the meantime, my love, with deepest gratitude, every word of this is for you.

Also by Felicia Luna Lemus and available from Akashic Books

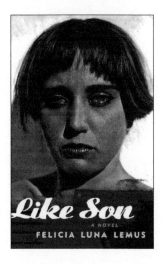

LIKE SON

238 pages, trade paperback original, $15.95

Finalist for the 2008 Ferro-Grumley
Award for LGBT Fiction

"Felicia Luna Lemus is a literary alchemist."
—Vendela Vida, author of
The Diver's Clothes Lie Empty

"*Like Son* is one terrific read."
—Eileen Myles, author of *Cool for You*

"[A] powerfully written chronicle of
love." —*Booklist*

"*Like Son* is a love story that, like a psychic's trick, leaves nothing un-
bent: not gender, not culture north and south of the border, not time,
or friendship, not even love itself. Don't try to understand how it hap-
pens; just watch, and be amazed."
—Paul La Farge, author of *The Night Ocean*

"Chaos and fate are hopelessly intertwined in this exuberant second
novel . . . Lemus doesn't waste a word in this smart, never sentimental
novel."
—*Publishers Weekly*

"[A] sweet song of a story." —Michelle Tea, author of *Against Memoir*